Low glycemic index 2

Delicious Recipes for a Healthy Life

SUMMARY :

- 6. Vegetables and vegetable chickpeas
- 7. Endives with chicken breast au gratin
- **Dessert and snack ideas**
- 1. Lemon and aqua faba cake
- 2. Banana and chocolate smoothie
- 3. Pear and cinnamon smoothie
- 4. Arbutus compote
- 5. Sweet oat okara pancakes
- 6. Oatmeal cookies
- 7. Flan without dough
- 8. Roasted fruits with spices
- 9. Buckwheat and banana cake
- 10. Apple-peanut butter smoothie with chia seeds
- 11. Apple Slices with Peanut Butter
- 12. Peanut Butter Energy Balls
- **Menu idea for low glycemic index meals**

Presentation of the Author: Ig Bas

I am a passionate author and a strong advocate for health and wellness. After profoundly transforming my own lifestyle through a low-glycemic diet, I now share my knowledge and experiences through books.

In this second book, "Low Glycemic Index Food: Delicious Recipes for a Healthy Life", I further deepen my commitment to a balanced diet. Building on my first successful experience, I continue to explore the benefits of tasty, accessible and health-friendly cuisine.

His Journey

Following medical tests revealing worrying blood sugar levels, I made the decision to radically change my lifestyle. By eliminating sugar and adopting a diet focused on ingredients with a low glycemic index, by walking daily and swimming in the pool or sea, I not only lost weight, but I also regained energy and energy. remarkable well-being. My first book has already inspired many people to do the same, and this new volume is a continuation of this approach

What You Will Find in This Book

- Practical advice: Tips on how to integrate these recipes into your daily life and improve your health without giving up the pleasure of eating well.

- Nutritional Guides: A detailed explanation of what the glycemic index is and why it is crucial to maintaining good health.

- Tasty Recipes: Easy-to-prepare recipes, ranging from main dishes to desserts, which promote diversity and taste while remaining faithful to the principles of a low glycemic index diet.

Ig Bas dedicates this book to all those who are looking for a healthier lifestyle. With a motivating approach and accessible advice, he demonstrates once again that simple food choices can have a huge impact on our overall well-being.

Follow Ig Bas on this culinary adventure and discover how a change in perspective on food can transform your life.

Practical Tips for Incorporating Low Glycemic Index Recipes

1. Plan your Meals:
   - Set aside time each week to plan your meals. This will allow you to choose low glycemic index recipes and make a shopping list accordingly, thus avoiding impulsive choices.

2. Prepare in Advance:
   - Cook in large quantities and freeze portions of your favorite recipes. This will make it easier on days when you don't have time to cook.

3. Use Basic Ingredients:
   - Stock low-glycemic index foods in your kitchen, such as legumes, whole grains, fresh vegetables and nuts. Having these ingredients on hand will inspire you to prepare healthy meals.

4. Edit Your Favorite Recipes:
   - Adapt your classic recipes by replacing high glycemic index ingredients with healthier alternatives.

For example, use almond flour instead of white flour or opt for natural sweeteners instead of refined sugar.

5. Eat Mindfully:
   - Take the time to savor every bite of your meals. This will not only help you enjoy the flavors, but also help you better regulate your appetite.

6. Incorporate Vegetables into All Your Meals:
   - Add vegetables to every dish, whether salads, soups or main dishes. They are high in fiber and nutrients while having minimal impact on your blood sugar.

7. Hydrate Properly:
   - Drink plenty of water throughout the day (1.5 liters to 2 liters of water/day). Replace sugary drinks with sugar-free infusions or flavored waters to satisfy your flavor cravings.

8. Make Healthy Snacks:
   - Prepare healthy snacks like nuts, veggie sticks with hummus, or fresh fruit. This can help you avoid unhealthy snacking.

9. Listen to Your Body:
   - Learn to recognize hunger and fullness signals. Eat when you're actually hungry and stop when you're full.

10. Share Your Meals:
   - Invite your family or friends to share a meal prepared using low glycemic index recipes. This will make the dining experience even more enjoyable!

By integrating these practical tips into your daily life, you can easily adopt a low glycemic index diet without sacrificing the pleasure of eating well. Taking care of your health can be a delicious and rewarding experience!

What is the Glycemic Index and Why is it Crucial for Health?

What is the glycemic index?
The glycemic index (GI) is a measurement that ranks foods based on their impact on blood glucose (sugar) levels after consumption. Foods with a high glycemic index (like white bread, sweets, and processed foods) cause a rapid rise in blood sugar, while those with a low glycemic index (like vegetables, legumes, and whole grains) cause a more rapid rise. slow and more stable blood sugar level.

Here is how GI is generally classified:
- Low GI: 0 to 55
- Moderate GI: 56 to 69
- High GI: 70 and above

Why is the Glycemic Index crucial for Health?

1. Blood Sugar Control:
  - Foods with a low glycemic index help stabilize blood glucose levels, reducing the risk of sudden spikes and drops in blood sugar. This is especially important for people who have diabetes or are looking to prevent this disease.

2. Weight Management:
  - Low GI foods are generally higher in fiber and nutrients, which promotes satiety. This can help reduce cravings and snacking, making long-term weight management easier.

3. Sustainable Energy:
  - Consuming foods with a low glycemic index helps maintain a constant energy level throughout the day. This avoids fatigue linked to blood sugar fluctuations often caused by high GI foods.

4. Prevention of Chronic Diseases:
  - A diet rich in foods with a low glycemic index is associated with a reduced risk of developing chronic

diseases, such as heart disease, obesity, and certain types of cancer. This is due to overall improved metabolic health and reduced inflammation in the body.

5. Better Food Quality:
   - Often, low GI foods, such as fruits, vegetables, nuts and whole grains, are less processed and contain more essential nutrients. By integrating these foods into your diet, you promote optimal nutritional balance.

Nutritional Tips for Incorporating the Low Glycemic Index into Your Diet:

- Choose Whole Grains: Opt for whole grains and pastas rather than refined products.
- Consume Legumes: Include lentils, beans and chickpeas in your dishes to increase the protein and fiber content.
- Favor fruits and vegetables: Favor whole fruits rather than juices and choose a variety of fresh vegetables at each meal.
- Limit Added Sugars: Avoid processed foods high in added sugars and learn to read food labels.
- Balance your meals: Combine low GI carbohydrates with lean proteins and healthy fats for prolonged satiety.

By paying more attention to the glycemic index of your foods, you can make more informed dietary decisions, improve your overall health, and experience a more flavorful and satisfying diet.

Here are some tips and tricks to help you lower the glycemic index of your meals and better manage your blood sugar:

Tips and Tricks for Lowering the Glycemic Index

1. Prefer Whole Foods:
   - Choose unprocessed foods, such as vegetables, whole fruits, whole grains and named proteins. Avoid refined and processed foods that often contain added sugars.

2. Opt for Whole Grains:
   - Replace white bread, white rice and refined pasta with their wholemeal versions (wholemeal bread, brown rice, whole wheat pasta). These foods have a lower glycemic index and are also higher in fiber.

3. Include Protein and Healthy Fats:
   - Add protein sources (like lean meats, fish, eggs, legumes) and healthy fats (like avocado, nuts, olive oil)

to your meals. This slows the digestion and absorption of carbohydrates, reducing blood sugar spikes.

4. Eat Foods Rich in Fiber:
   - Increase your fiber intake by including vegetables, fruits, seeds and legumes in your diet. Fiber helps slow the absorption of carbohydrates and stabilize blood sugar levels.

5. Don't Skip Meals:
   - Eat regularly throughout the day to avoid drops in blood sugar that can cause sugar cravings. Balanced meals and healthy snacks keep your energy levels stable.

6. Use Natural Sweeteners:
   -If you need a little sweetness, opt for natural sweeteners like stevia or maple syrup in small amounts, rather than refined sugar.

7. Choose Cooking Methods:
   - Prepare your food by steaming, baking, spit or grilled, instead of frying. These methods help preserve nutrients and avoid added fats that can negatively influence your blood sugar.

8. Avoid Eating in Speed:
  - Take the time to eat and savor every bite. This helps to better regulate appetite and avoid consuming too many carbohydrates in a short time.

9. Focus on Raw Vegetables:
  - Eating vegetables raw or lightly cooked (such as steamed) can help lower the glycemic index of the foods you eat. Long cooking can increase the GI of certain foods.

10. Pay Attention to Portions:
  - Limit your portion sizes, especially foods with a higher glycemic index. Even healthy foods can impact your blood sugar if eaten in excess.
11. Hydrate yourself:
  - Drink plenty of water and avoid sugary drinks. Hydration helps maintain a healthy metabolism and regulate sugar cravings.

12. Add Spices:
   - Certain spices like cinnamon, turmeric and ginger can help regulate blood sugar levels. Incorporate them into your dishes to add flavor and added benefits.

By implementing these tips and tricks, you can change your diet to favor healthy, low-glycemic choices, helping to stabilize your blood sugar and improve your overall well-being.

Here is a list of healthy protein sources you can incorporate into your diet to help stabilize your blood sugar and improve your health:

Sources of Protein to Consume

1. Lean meats:
    - Chicken (breast, thigh without skin)
    - In religion
    - Lean beef (like filet or striploin)
    - Pork (filet mignon)

2. Fish and Seafood:
    - Salmon (rich in omega-3)
    - Trout
    - Sardines
    - Mackerel
    - Shrimp

3. Eggs:
    - Whole eggs or egg whites, an excellent source of high-quality protein.

4. Legumes:
   - Lenses
   - Chickpeas
   - Black beans
   - Red beans
   - Beans (such as white beans or wild beans)

5. Dairy Products:
   - Greek yogurt (preferable without added sugar)
   - Cottage cheese
   - Milk (or protein-enriched vegetable milk)

6. Nuts and Seeds:
   - Almonds
   - Cashew nuts
   - Nut
   - Chia seeds
   - Flax seeds
   - Sunflower seeds

7. Meat Substitutes:
   - Tofu (rich in protein and versatile)
   - Tempeh (fermented soy source with better
digestibility)

- Seitan (made from wheat gluten, rich in protein)

8. Whole Cereals:
   - Quinoa (considered a whole grain and good source of protein)
   - Oats (especially whole oats)

Tips for Getting More Protein into Your Diet:

- Add legumes to your salads and soups.
- Prepare omelettes with vegetables and spices for breakfast.
- Choose snacks based on Greek yogurt with fruits and nuts.
- Opt for fish at least twice a week.
- Explore dishes based on tofu or tempeh (food product made from fermented soybeans, it is a rich source of protein, known for its many nutritional benefits) by marinating and grilling them.

By incorporating these protein sources into your diet, you not only promote better blood sugar control, but you also provide your body with the nutrients needed for optimal health.

Here are some ideas for tasty starters adapted to a low glycemic index (low GI)

Here is a recipe for quinoa and vegetable salad with precise proportions for each ingredient:

Quinoa and vegetable salad

Ingredients for 4 people:

- 200 g of raw quinoa or bulgur (around 600 g cooked)
- 1 red pepper, diced
- 1 yellow pepper, diced
- 1 green pepper, diced
- 1 cucumber, diced
- 200 g cherry tomatoes, cut in half
- 1 avocado, diced (optional)
- 3 tablespoons of lemon juice (about 1 to 2 lemons)
- 4 tablespoons of olive oil
- Salt and pepper to taste

- 1/2 cup fresh herbs (parsley or cilantro), chopped

Preparation :

1. Cooking the quinoa:
   - Rinse the quinoa under cold water to remove its bitterness.
   - In a saucepan, bring 600 ml of water to the boil (or 2 parts water for 1 part quinoa).
   - Add the quinoa and a pinch of salt. Reduce the heat to medium-low, cover and simmer for about 15 minutes, or until the water is absorbed and the quinoa is tender.
   - Remove from the heat, let sit for 5 minutes, then fluff with a fork.

2. Preparation of vegetables:
   - While the quinoa is cooking, prepare the peppers, cucumber, cherry tomatoes and avocado (optional). Put them in a large bowl.

3. Assemble the salad:
   - Add the cooked and cooled quinoa to the vegetables in the bowl.

- Drizzle with lemon juice and olive oil. Season with salt
and pepper.
   - Add the chopped fresh herbs and mix gently to combine all
the ingredients well.

4. Serve:
   - Refrigerate the salad for about 30 minutes before serving
to allow the flavors to blend, or serve immediately.

 Suggestions :
- You can add other ingredients according to your taste, such
as olives, radishes, nuts or seeds for more crunch.
- This salad is perfect for a light meal, as a side dish or for a
picnic.

Enjoy your quinoa and vegetable salad!

Bulgur salad with vegetables

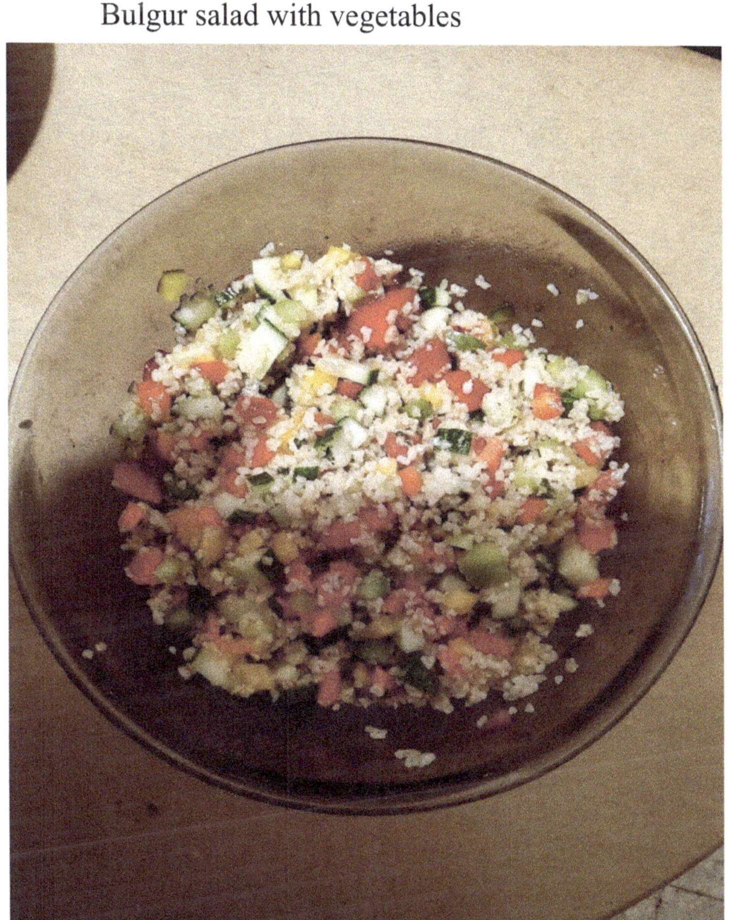

Chickpea quinoa balls

Amazing ! This quinoa and chickpea recipe is better than meat! Protein-rich chickpea recipe! [Vegan]

Ingredients :
240 g canned chickpeas
90g (1/2 cup) rinsed quinoa
60 g chopped walnuts
1 onion
2 cloves of garlic
2 pepper halves 1 red and 1 yellow or 1 whole of your choice

Instructions:
 1st Quinoa Cooking:
 Rinse the quinoa well and place it in a saucepan with water (2:1 water/quinoa ratio).
 Cook for about 15 minutes until fully cooked and bubbly. Drain excess water and set aside.

2nd Prepare the chickpeas:
Drain the chickpeas and mash them with a fork in a
large bowl. You can also use a food processor to get a
smoother texture.

3rd Brown the onion and garlic:
In a lightly oiled pan, sauté the sliced onion over
medium heat until soft (about 3-4 minutes).
Add the minced garlic and cumin seeds and cook for
another minute until fragrant.

4. Mix the ingredients:
To the bowl with the chickpea puree, add the cooked
quinoa, sautéed onion and garlic, ground walnuts,
breadcrumbs (or chickpea crumbs), and nutritional yeast
(if using).

Season with sweet peppers, dried herbs, Korean chili
flakes (optional), and salt to taste.
Mix everything well until all the ingredients are well
combined.

5. Form the balls:
Preheat the oven to 350°F (180°C).

Lightly grease or line a baking sheet with parchment
paper.
Using your hands, form 30 g balls of the mixture and
place them on the prepared baking sheet.
Spray or lightly brush the balls with oil to help them
crisp up in the oven.

6. Cook:
Bake for 15 minutes or until the balls are golden brown
and slightly crispy on the outside.

Presentation suggestions:
With sauce: Serve with dairy-free yogurt, cream or spicy
tomato sauce.

With salad: Serve with a fresh green salad for a
complete and nutritious meal.
Snack or appetizer: Enjoy as a protein-rich snack or as
an appetizer with sauce.

quinoa/bulgur meatballs, chickpeas, peppers

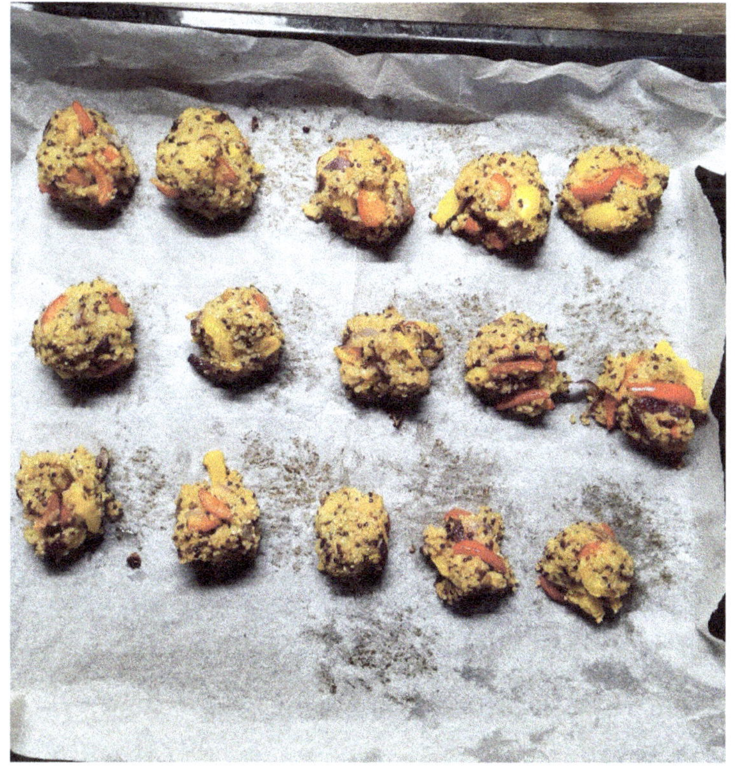

Cooking tips:

Quinoa: Make sure the quinoa is well drained to avoid excess moisture in the mixture.

Texture: For a smoother mixture, use a food processor to grind the chickpeas and blend the ingredients.

Seasoning: Adjust seasoning to taste; add additional chili flakes for added heat or increase dried herbs for more flavor.

Nutritional benefits:
High in protein: Chickpeas, quinoa and nuts are an excellent source of plant-based protein.

Rich in fiber: promotes healthy digestion and keeps you fuller for longer.
B Vitamins: Nutritional yeast provides cheesy flavor while adding valuable B vitamins.

Dietary information:

Gluten-free: Use chickpea crumbs or gluten-free breadcrumbs.

Dairy-Free and Vegan: This recipe is naturally dairy-free and 100% plant-based.

Storage:

Refrigerate: Store leftovers in an airtight container in the refrigerator for up to 3 days.
Reheating: Heat them in the oven at 180°C (350°F) for 10 to 12 minutes to maintain their crispness.

Why you will love this recipe:

Easy to prepare: With simple steps and ingredients, it is very easy to prepare.

Nutritious and filling: a healthy, protein-rich alternative to traditional meatballs.

Versatile: Serve them in different ways for different meals.

Conclusion:

These roasted chickpea and quinoa balls are a delicious and nutritious addition to your meal rotation. Whether you're looking for a healthy main course or a healthy snack, these protein-rich portions will satisfy you. Try them with your favorite sauce and enjoy a burst of flavor and nutrition!
Source of protein.

Here is a simple and delicious recipe for yogurt sauce, whether savory or sweet. This sauce is light and full of flavor, perfect to accompany your pancakes.

Yogurt Sauce

Ingredients :
- 250 g of natural yogurt (natural, Greek or plant-based)
- 1 tablespoon of lemon juice
- 1 clove of garlic, minced or pressed (optional)
- 1 teaspoon of cumin powder or paprika (adjust according to your preference)
- 1 tablespoon of olive oil
- Salt and pepper to taste
- Fresh herbs (such as mint, parsley or coriander), finely chopped (optional)

Instructions :

1. Mix the ingredients:
   - In a bowl, add the natural yogurt, lemon juice, minced garlic, cumin (or paprika), and olive oil.
   - Mix well until you obtain a homogeneous consistency.
2. Season:
   - Add salt and pepper to taste. If desired, also add chopped fresh herbs for a fresher taste.

3. Refrigerate:
   - Let the sauce sit in the refrigerator for about 15 to 30 minutes before serving. This will allow the flavors to blend together.

4. Serve:
   - Serve the yogurt sauce with your hot low igs. It can also be used as a dip for other dishes

Variants:

- Spices: You can experiment with other spices like curry, thyme or dill.
- Additions: For a smoother sauce, add a little cream cheese or crumbled feta.

This yogurt sauce is not only easy to make, but it also adds a refreshing and tasty touch to your patties. Enjoy your food !

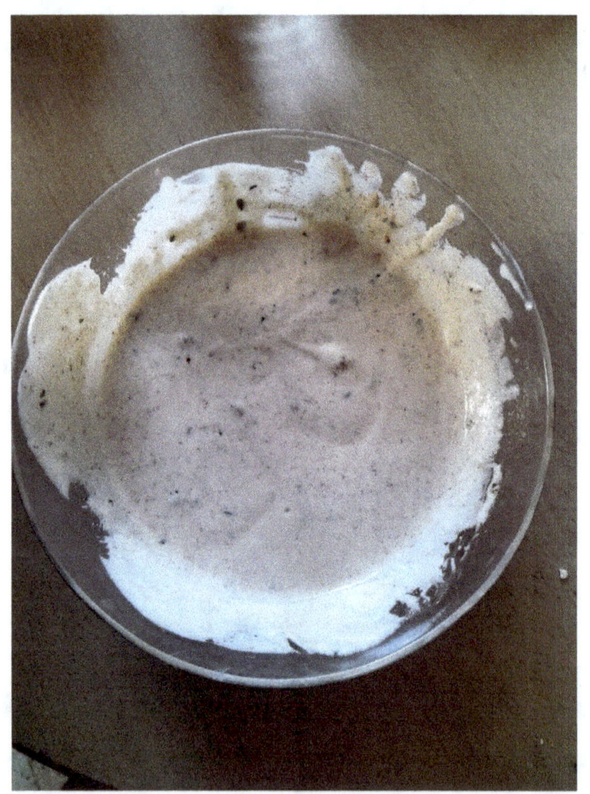

Yogurt sauce is a great accompaniment, but it is important to store it properly to maintain its freshness and food safety. Here are some tips for conservation:

Storing Yogurt Sauce

1. Refrigeration
   - Duration: Yogurt sauce generally keeps in the refrigerator for 3 to 5 days.
   - Packaging: Place the sauce in an airtight container to avoid absorbing odors from other foods in the refrigerator. A glass jar or closed plastic container is ideal.

2. Freezing (optional)
   - If you want to keep the sauce longer, you can freeze it. However, the texture may change slightly after thawing.
   - Duration: In the freezer, the sauce can be kept for up to 2 months.

   - Packaging:
Use an airtight container or freezer bags. Leave some room for the yogurt to expand as it freezes.

3. Defrosting

 -To use frozen sauce, thaw it in the refrigerator for a few hours or overnight. Avoid thawing at room temperature to reduce the risk of bacteria growth.

4. Signs of expiry

 - Before consuming the yogurt sauce, check for signs of spoilage, such as an unpleasant odor, unusual texture or the presence of mold. If you have any doubts, it is best not to consume it.

Additional Tips
- Avoid contamination: always use clean utensils to serve the sauce to avoid contaminating the rest of the mixture.
- Spices and herbs: If you are adding fresh herbs or ingredients that can go bad quickly, it is best to add them just before serving the sauce.

By following these recommendations, you will be able to enjoy your yogurt sauce while ensuring its freshness and safety.

Here are some ideas for low glycemic index dishes (low GI both with and without meat or fish:

Chicken Curry and Vegetables

- Ingredients :
  - 500 g of chicken breast or thighs, cut into pieces
  - 1 onion, chopped
  - 2 carrots, cut into slices
  - 1 zucchini, diced
  - 400 ml of coconut milk
  - 2 tablespoons of curry paste (or to taste)
  - Olive oil
  - Salt and pepper

- instruction :
  1. In a pan, heat the olive oil and fry the onion until translucent.
  2. Add the chicken and cook until golden brown

3. Add the vegetables, curry paste, then coconut milk.
Let simmer for 20 minutes. Serve hot.

Chicken curry with vegetables (here with more liquid)

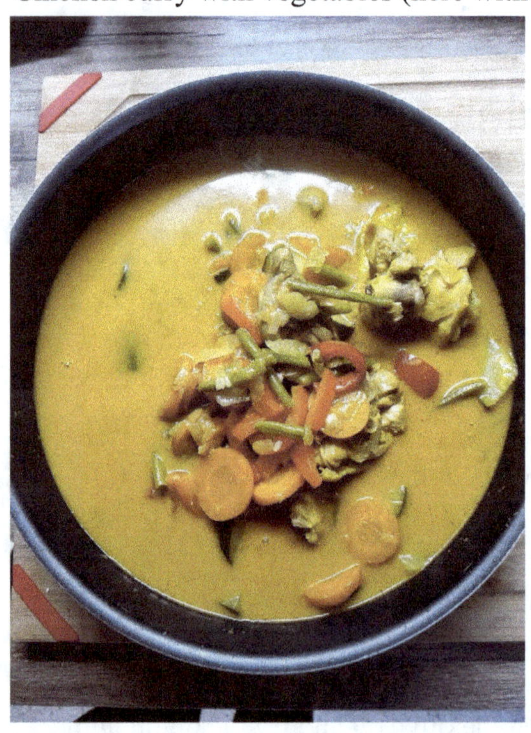

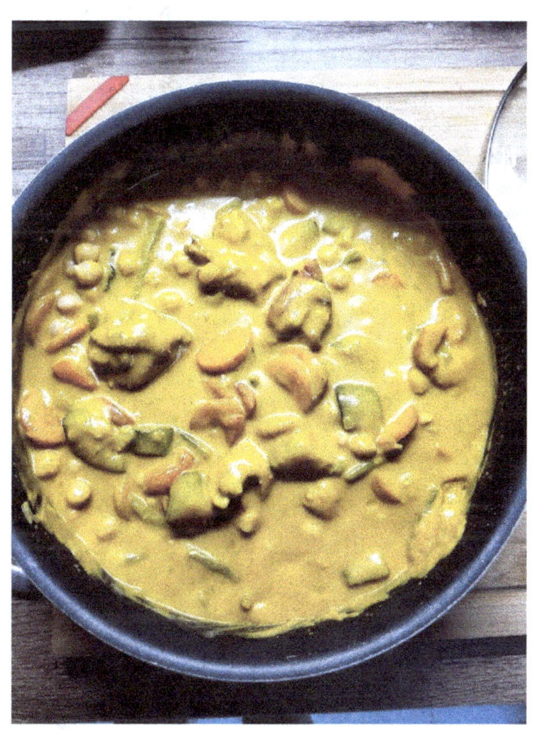

same recipe with chickpeas

Here is a delicious recipe for stuffed eggplant with a low glycemic index. This recipe uses healthy, flavorful ingredients to create a hearty and nutritious dish.

Low GI Stuffed Eggplant

Ingredients for 4 people
- 2 large eggplants
- 200 g of lean ground meat (beef, chicken, or turkey) or vegetable proteins such as crumbled tofu
- 1 medium onion, chopped
- 2 cloves of garlic, minced
- 1 red green pepper, diced
- 200 g crushed tomatoes (canned or fresh)
- 1 teaspoon of Provence herbs (or other herbs such as thyme or basil)
- 50 g grated cheese (optional, for garnish)
- Salt and pepper to taste
- 2 tablespoons of olive oil

- Optional: 1 grated zucchini or other vegetables of your choice
- Fresh parsley for garnish

Instructions :

1. Preheating the oven:
   - Preheat your oven to 180°C (350°F).

2. Preparation of eggplants:
   - Wash the eggplants and cut them in half lengthwise. Using a spoon, carefully remove the flesh to create boats. Reserve the eggplant flesh in a bowl.

3. Cooking the stuffing:
   - In a large skillet, heat the olive oil over medium heat. Add the chopped onion and minced garlic. Fry until translucent.
   - Add the ground meat (or tofu) and cook until browned and cooked through. If you are using additional vegetables like zucchini, add them at this time to cook.
   - Incorporate the reserved eggplant flesh, the diced pepper and the crushed tomatoes. Add the Provence

herbs, salt and pepper. Simmer for about 5-10 minutes, until well mixed and the meat is cooked.

4. Stuff the eggplants:
   - Fill each eggplant half with the stuffing mixture, packing lightly.

5. Baking:
   - Place the stuffed eggplants in a baking dish. If desired, sprinkle grated cheese on top. Add a little water to the bottom of the dish to help keep the eggplants moist while cooking.
   - Bake for about 25 to 30 minutes, or until the eggplants are tender and the top is lightly browned.

6. Garnish:
   - Before serving, sprinkle with chopped fresh parsley to add color and freshness.

Suggestions :
- Variations: You can replace the meat with legumes (like lentils) for a vegetarian version.
- Accompaniment: Serve with a green salad or quinoa to complete the meal.

These stuffed eggplants are not only delicious, but also healthy and satisfying. Enjoy this tasty and nourishing dish!

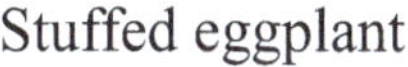

Stuffed eggplant

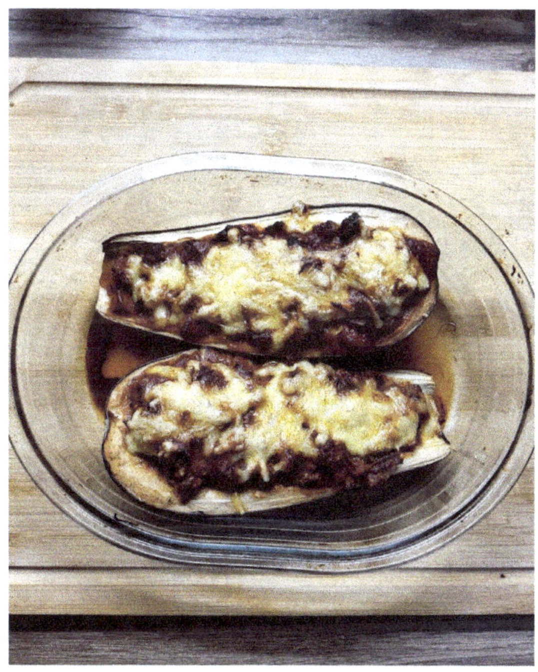

Spiced Fish Balls

- Ingredients: approximately 2 people
  - 300 g of white fish filet (cod, pollack, etc.)
  - 1 egg
  - 1 tablespoon of almond or coconut flour
  - 1 teaspoon of cumin powder
  - 1 teaspoon of paprika
  - Salt and pepper
  - Olive oil for cooking

- Instruction :

1. Mix the fish with the egg, flour, spices, salt and pepper until you obtain a homogeneous paste.

2. Form balls and cook them in a pan with a little olive oil until they are golden brown on each side. Serve with yogurt sauce and vegetables.

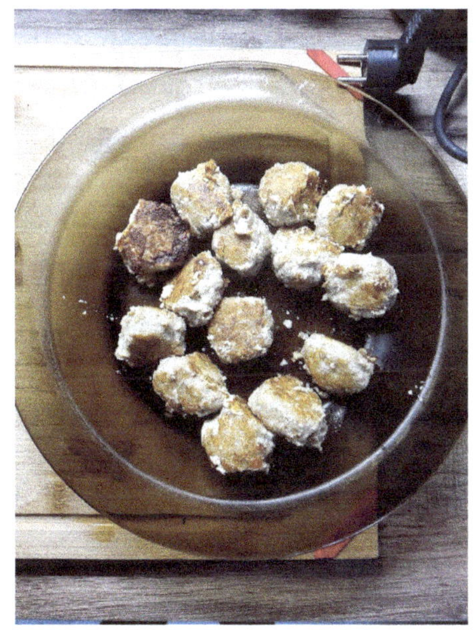

oatmeal fish balls

If you're looking to replace almond flour in spiced fish balls, there are several options that can maintain the texture and flavor. Here are some alternatives:

1. Coconut Flour
- Description: Coconut flour is an excellent alternative, particularly for low GI recipes. It's high in fiber and protein, but fluid absorption is higher, so use a little less than the amount of almond flour.
- Usage: Start with 1/4 of the required amount of almond flour and increase if necessary.

2. Chickpea Flour
- Description: Chickpea flour is rich in protein and fiber, with a slightly nutty taste, which goes well with fish balls.
- Use: Replace the almond flour with the same quantity of chickpea flour.

3. **Oatmeal**
- Description: Oatmeal has a moderate GI, but it is quite nutritious and can be used to bind ingredients in fish balls.
- Use: Use the same quantity as almond flour. Make sure it is gluten free if necessary.

4. **Whole Wheat Semolina (or Whole Wheat Flour)**
- Description: If gluten is not a problem, whole wheat semolina is a good option to give a pleasant consistency to the meatballs.
- Use: Replace with the same quantity as the almond flour.

5. **Buckwheat Flour**
- Description: High in protein and gluten-free, buckwheat flour has a slightly earthy taste, which can add an interesting touch to your dumplings.
- Use: Use the same quantity as almond flour.

6. **Panko or Wholemeal Bread Crumbs**

- Description: If you are looking for a crunchy texture, panko or wholemeal bread crumbs can work, although they are not specifically low GI.
- Use: Replace the almond flour with an equivalent quantity.

Another basic recipe for fish balls with spices

Ingredients: approximately 4 people
- 500 g of fish (such as cod or salmon), crumbled
- 1/2 cup almond flour or alternative
- 1 egg
- 1 tablespoon chopped fresh parsley
- 1 teaspoon of cumin powder
- 1 teaspoon of paprika
- 1 clove of garlic, minced
- Salt and pepper to taste
- Olive oil for cooking

Instructions :
1. In a large bowl, combine the flaked fish, flour (of your choice), egg, herbs, spices, garlic, salt and pepper.
2. Form balls with the mixture, rolling between your hands.
3. In a pan, heat a little olive oil over medium heat.
4. Cook the meatballs until golden brown on both sides (about 4-5 minutes per side).

5. Serve hot with yogurt sauce or tomato sauce.

These alternatives will allow you to make delicious fish balls while maintaining a good texture and an appreciable flavor. Enjoy your food !

Toulouse sausage with your lentil and carrot curry to make a complete and tasty meal. This will add an additional source of protein and enhance the flavors of the dish. Here's how you can incorporate sausage into the recipe:

Toulouse Sausage with Lentil and Carrot Curry

Ingredients: 4 people

- 2 to 3 Toulouse sausages, cut into rounds
- 200 g green or brown lentils (uncooked)
- 2 carrots, cut into slices
- 1 sweet potato (optional), diced
- 1 onion, chopped
- 2 cloves of garlic, minced
- 1 piece of fresh ginger (about 2 cm), grated
- 400 g crushed tomatoes (canned or fresh)

- 400 ml coconut milk (or unsweetened almond milk for
a lighter version)
- 2 tablespoons of olive oil or coconut oil
- 1 tablespoon of curry powder (or to taste)
- 1 teaspoon of cumin powder
- 1 teaspoon of turmeric powder
- Salt and pepper to taste
- Fresh coriander for garnish (optional)

Preparation :

1. Cooking lentils:
   - Rinse the lentils under cold water and drain them.

2. Preparation of the curry:
   - In a large pot or skillet, heat the olive oil or coconut
oil over medium heat.
   - Add the chopped onion and fry for about 5 minutes
until translucent.
   - Incorporate the garlic and ginger, then sauté for 1 to 2
minutes until they release their aromas.

3. Add vegetables:
 - Add the carrots and sweet potato (if using) to the pan. Cook for about 5 minutes, stirring.

4. Incorporation of lentils and spices:
 - Add the lentils, curry powder, cumin, turmeric, salt and pepper. Mix well to coat the vegetables and lentils with the spices.

5. Incorporation of tomatoes and coconut milk:
 - Pour the crushed tomatoes and coconut milk into the saucepan. Also add a glass of water (about 200 ml) to dilute the mixture.
 - Bring to the boil, then reduce the heat and simmer covered for about 25-30 minutes, or until the lentils and vegetables are tender. Stir occasionally and add a little water if the mixture becomes too thick.

6. Checking the seasoning:
 - Taste the curry and add salt, pepper or spices to taste.

1. Cooking sausages:
 - In the same pan you use for the curry, heat a little olive oil over medium heat.

- Add the Toulouse sausage slices and brown them for about 5 to 7 minutes until they are well cooked. Remove them and reserve them.

2. Incorporation of sausages:
   - After adding the crushed tomatoes and coconut milk, return the browned sausages to the pan. Make sure to mix well so everything is well coated in the curry mixture.

3. Mijotage :
   - Let everything simmer as directed, so that the flavors mix well and the sausages are well heated.

4. Service :
   - Serve the curry hot, garnished with fresh coriander if desired.

Suggestions :
- If you want the dish to be even more hearty, you can also add vegetables such as spinach or cauliflower during the preparation stages.
- This dish goes very well with quinoa, brown rice or even whole grain bread, depending on your preferences.

Enjoy this nourishing and comforting dish, which combines the good taste of lentils and vegetables with the richness of Toulouse sausage!

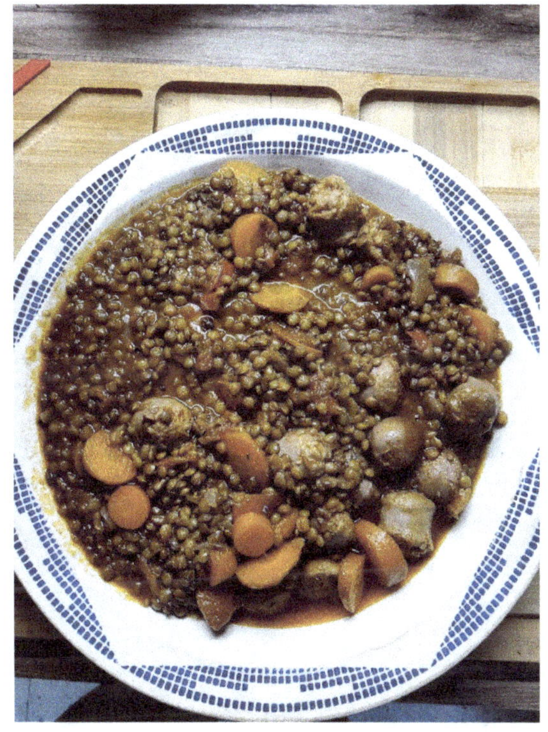

Toulouse Sausages with Lentil and Carrot Curry

A tasty and nourishing recipe with zucchini, chickpeas, carrots, broccoli and spices like curry and cumin. This dish can serve 2 to 3 people.

Curry vegetables and chickpeas

Ingredients :
- For the vegetable mixture:
  - 1 zucchini, diced
  - 1 carrot, peeled and cut into slices
  - 1 cup broccoli, cut into small pieces
  - 1 can (400 g) chickpeas, drained and rinsed
  - 1 onion, chopped
  - 2 tablespoons of olive oil
  - 2 cloves of garlic, chopped (optional)

- For the spices:
  - 1 teaspoon of curry powder
  - 1 teaspoon of cumin powder
  - 1/2 teaspoon of paprika (for a little color)

- Salt and pepper, to taste
- 1/2 cup vegetable broth or water (adjust to desired consistency)

Instructions :

1. Preparation of vegetables:
  - In a large skillet or saucepan, heat the olive oil over medium heat. Add the onions and fry them until they become translucent.
  - Add the garlic (if using) and sauté for another minute.

2. Add vegetables:
  - Add the carrots and mix well. Cook for about 5 minutes.
  - Add the zucchini and broccoli, then cook for another 3-4 minutes, stirring occasionally.

3. Incorporation of chickpeas:
  - Add the drained chickpeas to the pan. Mix well to incorporate the vegetables and chickpeas.

4. Add spices:
  - Add the curry, cumin, paprika, salt and pepper. Mix well to coat all the vegetables with the spices.
  - Pour in the vegetable stock or water to help cook and give a slightly creamy consistency. Simmer for 5 to 10 minutes over low heat, until the vegetables are tender.

5. Mixing (optional):
  - If you prefer a smooth texture, you can transfer the mixture to a blender and blend until you obtain the desired consistency. You can also add a little more water or broth if needed.

6. Taste and serve:
  - Taste and adjust seasoning if necessary. Serve hot, accompanied by rice, quinoa or pita bread if you wish.
 Conservation Tips:
- This dish keeps well in the refrigerator in an airtight container for 3 to 4 days.
- You can also freeze it for later use. Be sure to let it cool completely before freezing.

Variations :

- Feel free to add other vegetables you have on hand, such as peppers, spinach or mushrooms.
- For a spicy option, add some chili pepper or red pepper flakes.

Enjoy this comforting and nourishing dish!

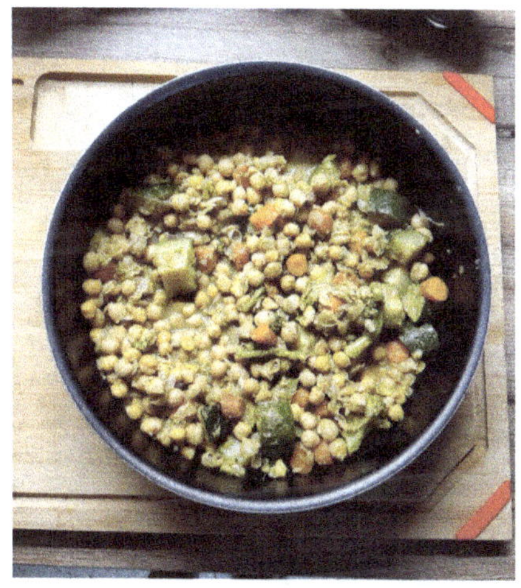

Chickpea curry with vegetables

Here is another recipe for endives with chicken breast au gratin, ideal for a tasty meal with a low glycemic index.

Endive with Chicken Breast Au Gratin

Ingredients (for 4 people):

- 4 endives
- 400 g of chicken breast (filets), cut into cubes
- 150 ml light crème fraîche (or soy cream for a lactose-free version)
- 100 g low-fat grated cheese (e.g. goat cheese or mozzarella)
- 1 tablespoon of olive oil
- 1 clove of garlic, minced
- 1 teaspoon of mustard (optional)
- Salt and pepper to taste
- Nutmeg (optional, for taste))

- Fresh parsley for garnish (optional)

Preparation :

1. Preparation of endives:
   - Preheat your oven to 200°C (390°F).
   - Cut the endives in half lengthwise and remove the bitter core. You can also blanch them in boiling salted water for 5 minutes, then drain them. This helps reduce bitterness.

2. Cooking the chicken:
   - In a pan, heat the olive oil over medium heat. Add the minced garlic and fry for a few minutes until golden.
   - Add the diced chicken and cook until they are nicely browned and cooked through (about 7 to 10 minutes). Season with salt, pepper and nutmeg (if using).
   - If you wish, incorporate the mustard to add a touch of taste.

3. Preparation of the sauce:
   - In a bowl, mix the crème fraîche with a little salt and pepper, and possibly a little nutmeg.

4. Assembling the dish:
   - In a gratin dish, place the endives flat. Spread the
chicken mixture over the endives.
   - Pour the cream over the endives and chicken, make
sure everything is well coated.
   - Sprinkle the grated cheese on top.

5. Baking:
   - Bake the dish for about 20 to 25 minutes, until the top
is nicely browned and the sauce is bubbling.

6. Service :
   - Serve hot, garnished with fresh parsley if desired.
This dish goes well with a green salad as an
accompaniment.

 Suggestions :
- You can also add spices like paprika or thyme to vary
the flavors.
- To increase the fiber content, you can serve this gratin
with a side of quinoa or legumes.

This endive gratin with chicken breast is both delicious and consistent with a low glycemic index diet. Enjoy

your food !

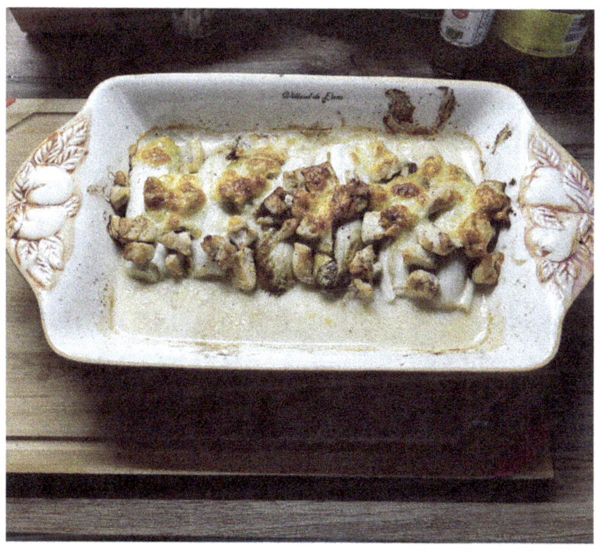

with coconut cream, nutmeg, mustard, gratinated with mozzarella

Here is 1 dessert or snack recipe

recipe based on aquafaba

Aqua Faba is the liquid left after cooking legumes, such as chickpeas. It is an excellent vegan substitute for egg whites and can be used in various recipes, including meringues, mousses or mayonnaise.

Definition of aqua faba:
- Aqua faba: This is the thick, viscous liquid obtained by cooking legumes such as chickpeas or using the preserving liquid from a can of legumes. It can be used as a substitute for egg whites in many recipes, especially for people who follow a vegan diet or have egg allergies.

Aqua Faba is a versatile and valuable alternative in vegan cooking, allowing you to create creamy and light dishes without animal products.

Lemon Cake with Aquafaba

Ingredients :
- 100 g oat flour (or low GI flour)
- 120 g of aquafaba (about 1/2 cup)
- 60 g of maple syrup or low GI sweetener
- Juice and zest of a lemon (around 30-40 g of juice)
- 10 g of baking powder
- A pinch of salt

Instructions :
1. Preheating: Preheat the oven to 180°C (350°F). Line a cake pan with parchment paper or lightly grease it.

2. Mix the dry ingredients: In a bowl, combine the oat flour, baking powder, and salt.

3. Prepare the wet mixture: In another bowl, beat the aquafaba with the maple syrup, lemon juice and lemon zest.

4. Combine the mixtures: Incorporate the wet mixture into the dry ingredients. Mix gently until you obtain a homogeneous paste.

5. Bake: Pour the batter into the prepared pan and smooth the top. Bake for 25 to 30 minutes, or until a toothpick inserted in the center comes out clean.

6. Cool and serve: Let the cake cool in the pan for 10 minutes before transferring it to a wire rack to cool completely. Serve plain or with a light icing made from yogurt or fruit compote.

Enjoy your food !

Aquafaba lemon cake

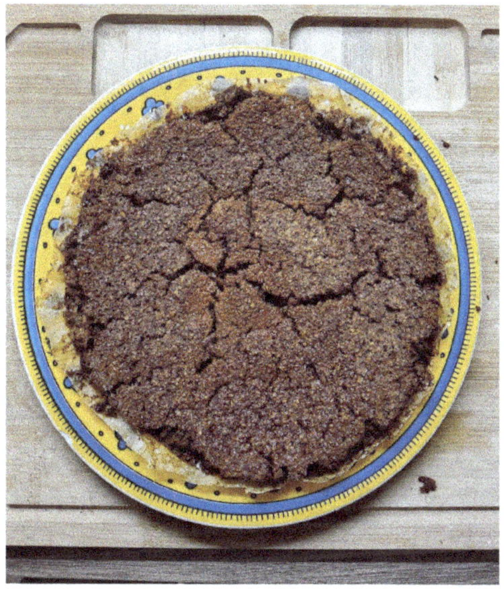

Here are some low GI smoothie recipes that are both delicious and nutritious. These smoothies use low GI ingredients to help you stay healthy while satisfying your cravings.

Chocolate-banana smoothie

Ingredients :
- 1 cup of almond milk or other unsweetened vegetable milk
- 1/2 banana (better if not too ripe for a low GI)
- 1 tablespoon of unsweetened cocoa powder
- 1 tablespoon of almond or nut butter
- 1 handful of spinach (for extra nutrients, optional)
- Ice cream (optional)

Instructions :
1. Mix all the ingredients in a blender.
2. Blend until smooth.
3. Adjust with a little more almond milk if necessary.

4. Serve chilled.

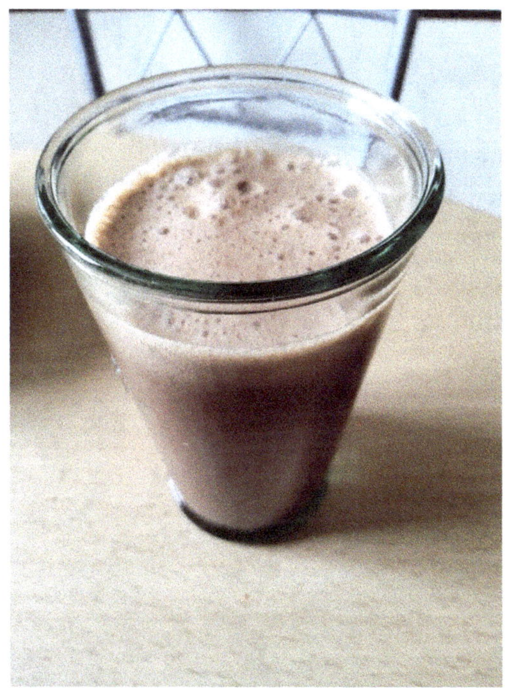

Chocolate/banana smoothie

Pear and Cinnamon Smoothie

Ingredients :
- 1 ripe pear, peeled and sliced
- 1 cup unsweetened almond milk
- 1 teaspoon of cinnamon
- 1 tablespoon of chia seeds
- 1/2 teaspoon vanilla (optional)
- Ice cream (optional)

Instructions :
1. Put all the ingredients in the blender.
2. Blend until smooth and creamy.
3. Enjoy immediately.

Remarks :
- You can always adjust the sweetness of your smoothies according to your tastes and needs by adding a natural sweetener (like a little honey, although it has a higher GI in small quantities).
- Smoothies can be customized a bit depending on what you have in your kitchen, but keep in mind to choose low GI fruits and vegetables to stay within the desired range.

Good smoothie !

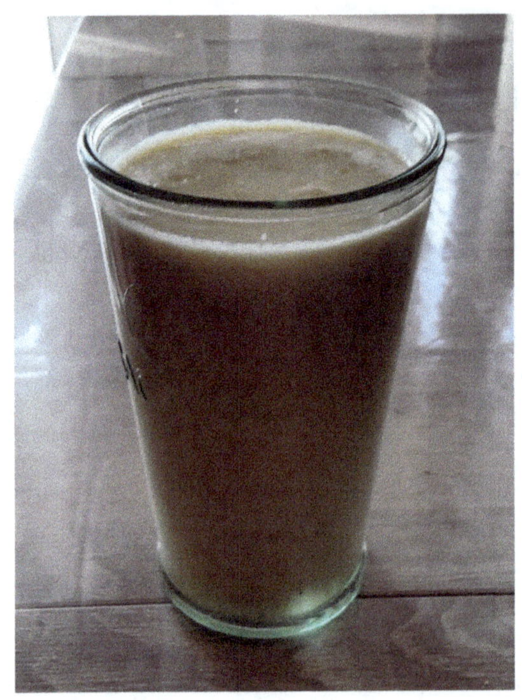

Pear/cinnamon

 It is also possible to make compote with arbutus, and it is an excellent idea to enjoy this delicious and lesser known fruit. Arbutus plants have a low glycemic index, which makes them compatible with a low glycemic index (low GI) diet. Here is a simple recipe for arbutus compote:

Arbutus compote

Ingredients :
- 500 g arbutus (ripe fruits)
- 1 to 2 tablespoons of agave syrup or a sweetener of your choice (adjust to taste)
- 1 teaspoon of lemon juice
- Optional: a pinch of cinnamon or vanilla to enhance the taste

Instructions :

1. Preparation of arbutus:
  - Wash the arbutus plants well to remove any impurities. Remove the stems and any pieces of leaves.

2. Cooking:
  - In a saucepan, put the arbutus, lemon juice and agave syrup. You can add a little water (about 2-3 tablespoons) to prevent it from sticking to the bottom of the pan.
  - Heat over medium heat, stirring occasionally, until the arbutus begins to break down and release its juice (about 10-15 minutes).

3. Mixing:
  - Once the fruit is well cooked, remove the pan from the heat. You can leave the compote chunky if you like or use a hand blender to get a smooth texture.

4. Taste adjustment:
  - Taste the compote and adjust the sweetness level by adding more agave syrup if necessary. If you chose to incorporate cinnamon or vanilla, add them at this point.

5. Cooling:

  - Let the compote cool before transferring it to an airtight jar or container. It will keep in the refrigerator for several days.

Suggestions :

- Use: This compote can be served with natural yogurt, on pancakes, or even as a topping for low GI desserts.
- Variations: You can add other fruits like apples or pears to vary the flavors.

Enjoy your arbutus compote, a delicious way to enjoy this fruit while keeping a low glycemic index!

Arbutus compote unfiltered

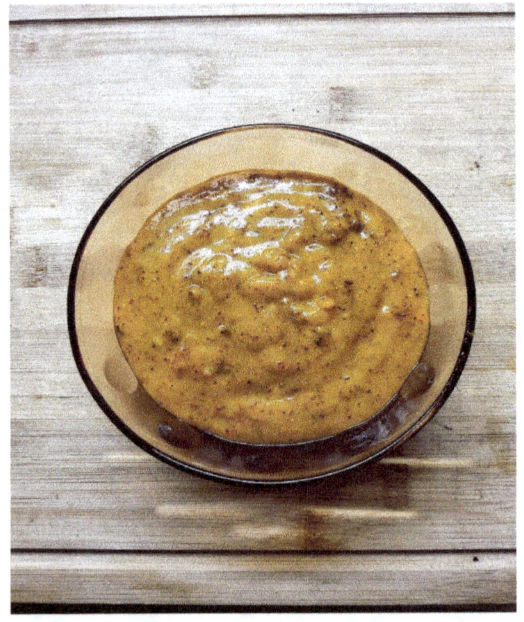

Filtered arbutus compote

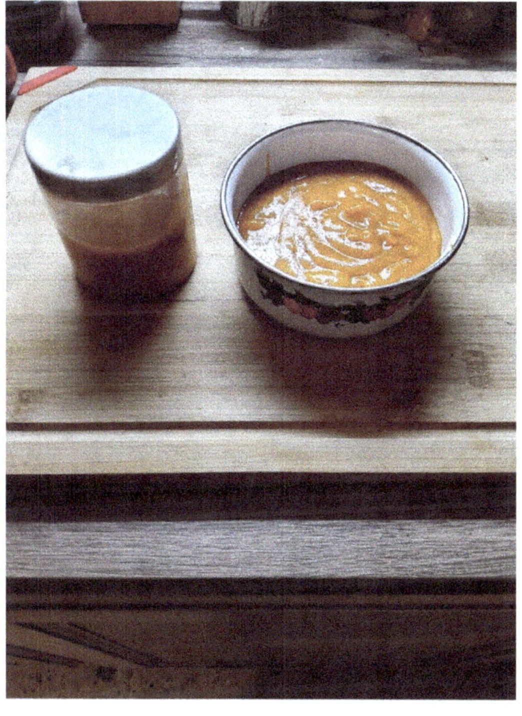

Sweet CAKES with Okara Oats

Ingredients :
- 150 g d'okara d'avoine
- 100 g oatmeal
- 2 ripe bananas, crushed
- 2 eggs
- 50 g of honey or maple syrup
- 1 teaspoon of cinnamon
- 1/2 teaspoon of baking soda
- A pinch of salt
- 50 g chopped walnuts or almonds (optional)

Instructions :

1. Prepare the mixture:
   - In a bowl, combine the oatmeal, oatmeal, mashed
bananas, eggs, honey, cinnamon, baking soda and salt.
Add nuts if desired.
   - Mix until you obtain a homogeneous consistency.

2. Cooking the pancakes:

- In a hot, lightly oiled pan, place spoonfuls of the mixture.

- Cook each patty for about 3-4 minutes on each side until golden brown.

3. Serve:

- Serve warm, possibly with a little yogurt or fresh fruit.

Oatmeal cookies, banana, compote instead of honey,

cinnamon, nutmeg, grapes

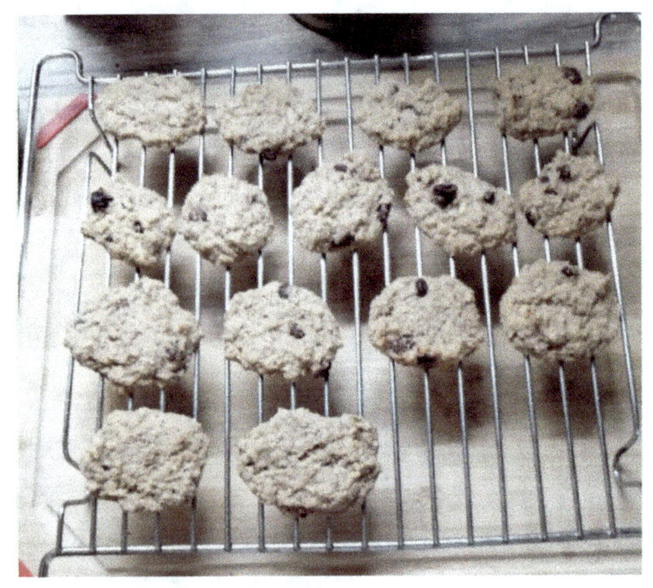

Here is a recipe for oatmeal cookies, oat flour and applesauce, with a touch of coconut, which has a low glycemic index. These cookies are healthy, delicious and easy to make!

Cookies with oatmeal

Ingredients

- For cookies:
  - 150 g oatmeal
  - 100 g of oat flour
  - 100 g applesauce without added sugar (or banana puree for a different taste)
  - 50 g melted coconut oil (or olive oil)
  - 50 g unsweetened grated coconut

  - 50 g of honey or agave syrup (adjust to taste, or use sweetener if desired)
  - 1 teaspoon of vanilla
  - 1/2 teaspoon of baking soda

- 1/2 teaspoon cinnamon (optional)
- 1 pinch of salt
- 50 g dark chocolate chips (optional, choose low GI chips)

Instructions

1. Preheat the oven:
   - Preheat your oven to 180°C (thermostat 6) and line a baking tray with baking paper.

2. Mixing dry ingredients:
   - In a large bowl, combine the oatmeal, oat flour, baking soda, cinnamon and salt.

3. Mixing wet ingredients:
   - In another bowl, mix the applesauce, melted coconut oil, honey (or agave syrup) and vanilla extract.

4. Incorporation of mixtures:
   - Add the wet mixture to the dry mixture and stir until well combined. If using chocolate chips, stir them in at this point.

5. Adding coconut:
  - Add the grated coconut and mix again until well incorporated.

6. Form the cookies:
  - Using a tablespoon, drop portions of dough onto the baking sheet, leaving a little space between each cookie.

7. Cooking:
  - Bake for about 12 to 15 minutes, or until the edges are lightly browned.

8. Cooling:
  - Let the cookies cool on the baking sheet for a few minutes, then transfer them to a wire rack to cool completely.

Enjoy your food !
These oatmeal, oatmeal, applesauce and coconut cookies are perfect for a healthy snack. They are soft, nourishing and delicious! Enjoy!

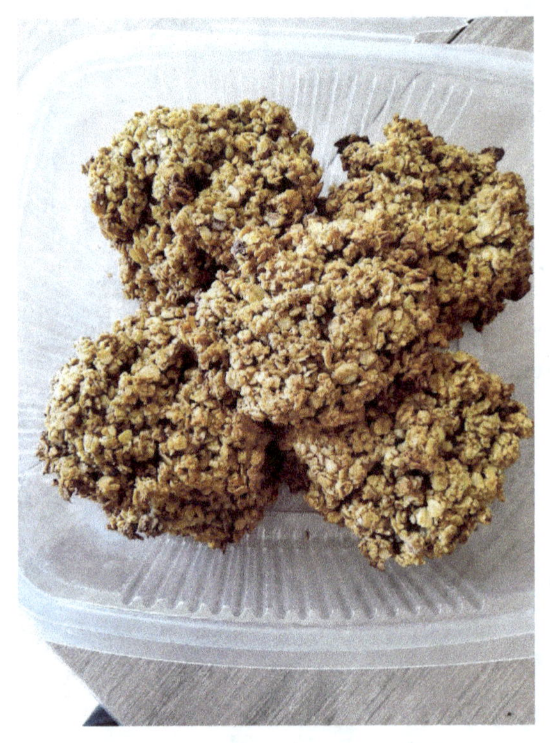

Almond cookies

Here is a pastry-free flan recipe with a low glycemic index. This flan is light and tasty, perfect for a guilt-free indulgent dessert.

Flan without Pastry with Low Glycemic Index

Ingredients :
- 500 ml of milk (or unsweetened almond milk for a lactose-free version)
- 3 eggs
- 50 g of agave syrup or maple syrup (or a low GI sweetener such as stevia or erythritol)
- 1 sachet of vanilla sugar or 1 teaspoon of vanilla extract
- 1 tablespoon of cornstarch (or potato starch for a gluten-free version)
- A pinch of salt

Instructions :

1. Preheating the oven:
   - Preheat your oven to 180°C (350°F).

2. Preparation of the mixture:
   - In a salad bowl, beat the eggs with the agave syrup
(or sweetener) and the vanilla. Then add the salt and
cornstarch, then mix well until you obtain a
homogeneous paste.

3. Add the milk:
   - Heat the milk in a saucepan over medium heat until
lukewarm, without boiling. Add the lukewarm milk to
the egg-sugar-mixture, and stir well.

4. Pour the mixture:
   - Pour the mixture into a flan mold or individual
ramekins, taking care not to overfill (the preparation will
swell a little during cooking).

5. Water bath:
   - Place the mold(s) in a baking dish half-filled with hot water (double boiler). This will help the flan cook evenly and stay soft.

6. Cooking:
   - Bake for about 30 to 40 minutes, or until the flan is firm to the touch and a knife comes out clean.

7. Cooling:
   - Let the flan cool to room temperature, then refrigerate it for at least 2 hours before eating.

 Suggestions :
- Light caramel: If you want a touch of caramel, you can make a light caramel with a sweetener like erythritol (heating it gently until you get a golden color) and pour it into the bottom of the molds before adding the preparation of the flan.
- Variations: You can add lemon or orange zest for a touch of freshness.

This flan is light, creamy and perfect for a low glycemic dessert. Enjoy it with fresh fruit for even more flavor!

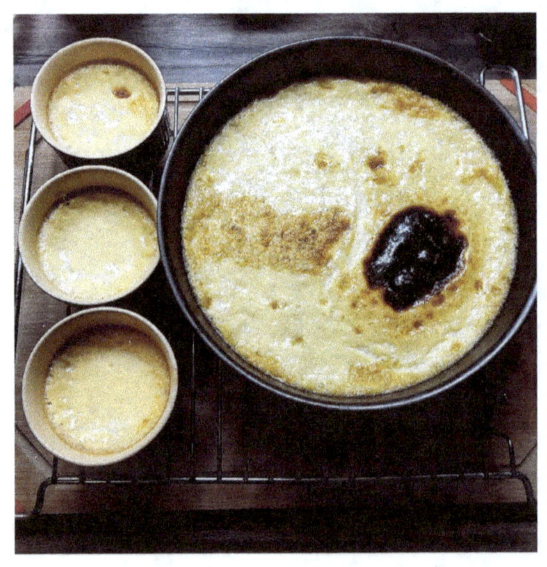

Flan without dough

Roasted Fruits with Spices

- Ingredients :
  - 2 apples or pears, cut into quarters
  - 1 tablespoon of olive oil
  - 1 teaspoon of cinnamon
  - 1/2 teaspoon nutmeg
  - Walnuts or almonds for crunch (optional)

- Preparation :

1. Preheat the oven to 200°C. Mix the fruit wedges with the olive oil and spices.

2. Place on a baking tray lined with parchment paper and roast for 20-25 minutes.

3. Serve warm, accompanied by natural yogurt or a scoop of sugar-free sorbet.

These desserts are not only deliciously satisfying, but they are also suitable for a low glycemic index diet. Enjoy it together with your family and friends!

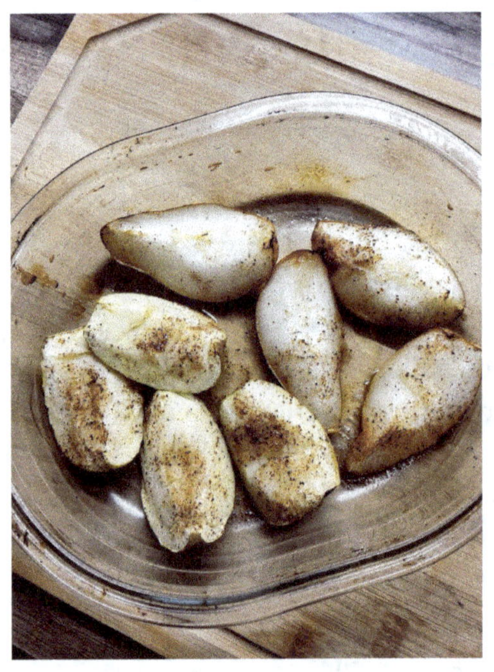

Roasted apples and pears, cinnamon and nutmeg

Make a cake using buckwheat flour, eggs, bananas, baking powder or baking powder, and grated coconut, replacing the sugar with honey or muscovado sugar. Here is a simple recipe suitable for foods with a low glycemic index:

Buckwheat and Banana Cake

Ingredients :
- 200 g buckwheat flour
- 2 eggs
- 2 ripe bananas (from which a sweet and moist taste comes)
- 1 small glass of vegetable milk of your choice
- 1 sachet of baking powder (or baking powder)
- 50 g grated coconut
- 2 to 3 tablespoons of honey or muscovado sugar (adjust to taste)
- 1 small pinch of salt
- A few nuts or seeds for crunch (optional)

Instructions :
1. Preheat Preheat your oven to 180°C (thermostat 6).
2. Preparation of the bananas In a large bowl, mash the bananas with a fork until you obtain a puree.
3. Mix wet ingredients: Add eggs and honey or muscovado sugar, milk to mashed banana, and mix well.
4. Add the dry ingredients to another bowl, mix together the buckwheat flour, baking powder, grated coconut and salt. Then incorporate this mixture into the wet ingredients.
5. Final mixture: Stir gently until ingredients are well combined. If desired, add nuts or seeds at this point.
6. Cooking:
Pour the batter into a cake pan previously greased or lined with parchment paper. Bake for about 30-35 minutes, or until a knife inserted in the center comes out clean.
7. Cooling: Let the cake cool for a few minutes in the mold, then unmold and let cool completely on a rack.

Advice :
- You can add spices like cinnamon or vanilla for more flavor.

- For a softer texture, you can replace part of the buckwheat flour with almond flour, if that suits you.

This cake is nourishing and ideal for a snack or dessert, while having a low glycemic index thanks to the use of the ingredients mentioned. Enjoy your food !

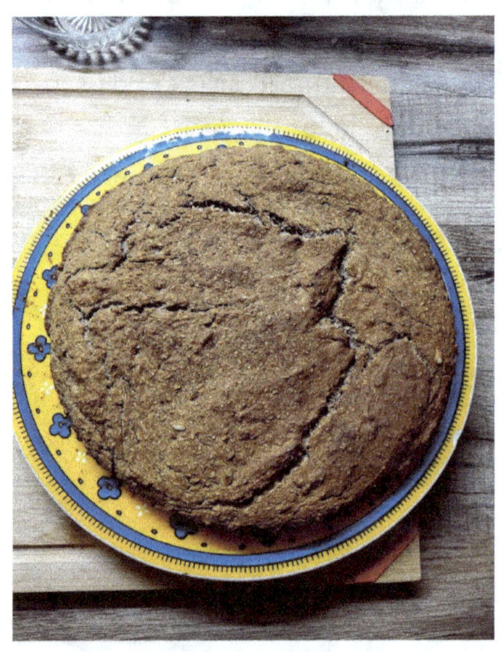

Buckwheat and banana cake

Peanut butter is a great ingredient for desserts and snacks that are both tasty and nutritious. Here are some creative ideas for integrating it into your recipes, while ensuring a low glycemic index:

Apple-Peanut Butter Smoothie with Chia Seeds

Ingredients :
- 1 cup of skim milk or 1/2 cup of cottage cheese
- 1 apple, cut into pieces (you can also use 1/2 orange or a pear if you prefer)
- 1 to 2 tablespoons of sugar-free peanut butter
- 1 tablespoon of chia seeds
- A little grated coconut (vanilla sugar, to your taste)
- A few ice cubes (optional, depending on the desired consistency)

Instructions :
1. In a blender, add the skimmed milk or cottage cheese.
2. Add the apple pieces, peanut butter, chia seeds and coconut.
3. Blend until smooth. If you want a colder texture, add ice cubes and blend again.
4. Taste and adjust the sweetness with vanilla sugar if necessary.
5. Pour into a glass and enjoy!

This smoothie is high in protein and fiber, ideal for a nutritious breakfast or snack. You can also customize this recipe to suit your tastes!

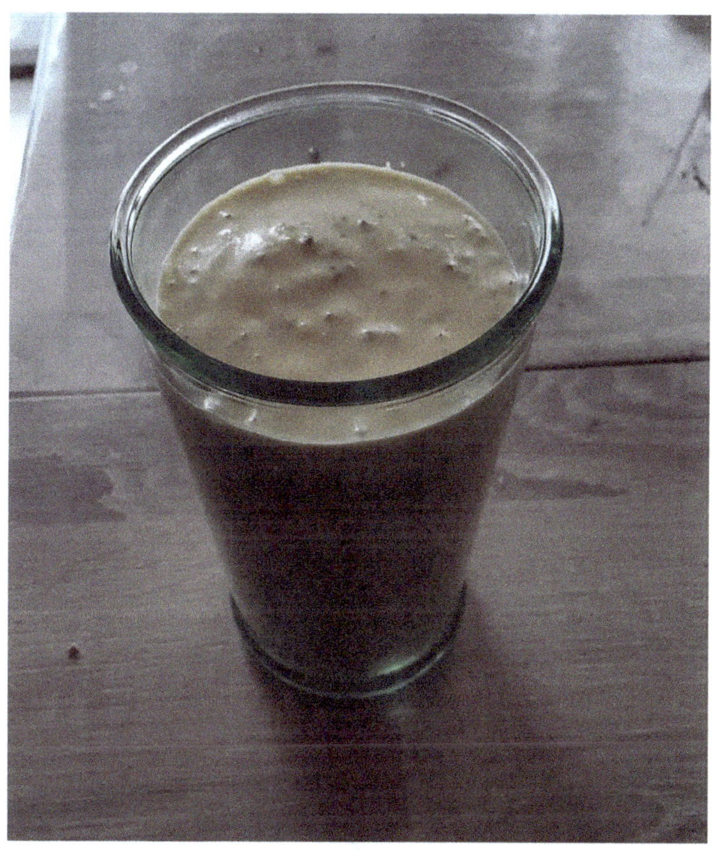

Smoothie 1/2 orange, cottage cheese, sugar-free peanut
butter, chia seeds, grated coconut

Apple Slices with Peanut Butter

A quick and easy way to enjoy peanut butter is to spread it on apple slices. This makes a crunchy and healthy snack! Add a pinch of cinnamon for even more flavor.

These ideas will allow you to use peanut butter deliciously in your desserts and snacks while maintaining a low glycemic index. Enjoy!

Peanut Butter Energy Balls

Ingredients
- 1 cup oatmeal (prefer quick-cooking oats for a finer texture)
- 1/2 cup natural peanut butter, no added sugar
- 1/4 cup honey or agave syrup (adjust to taste)
- 1/4 cup chia or flax seeds (for fiber)
- 1/4 cup chopped dark chocolate (at least 70% cocoa)
- Optional: grated coconut or dried fruit (no added sugar)

Instructions :
1. In a large bowl, mix all ingredients until well combined.
2. Form small balls with the mixture and place them on a baking sheet covered with parchment paper.
3. Refrigerate for at least 30 minutes before enjoying.
Store the balls in an airtight container in the refrigerator.

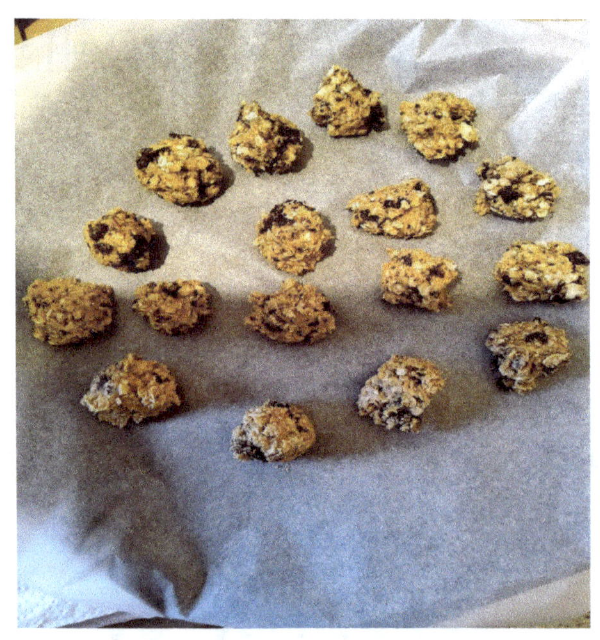

energy balls peanut butter, chocolate chips

Meal ideas for low glycemic index:

menu completely balanced and tasty while respecting a low glycemic index (low GI), here is an evaluation of the chosen dishes:

1. Spiced fish balls

- Benefits: Fish balls are rich in protein, which is excellent for satiety and health. Spices may also provide anti-inflammatory benefits.
- Suggestions: To keep the meal low GI, make sure to choose the ingredients carefully, especially the flour used to bind the meatballs, and avoid adding ingredients high in sugar.

2. Yogurt Sauce

- Benefits: Yogurt, especially plain yogurt without added sugar, is rich in protein and probiotics, which promotes digestive health.
- Suggestions: You can enrich the sauce with fresh herbs (like mint or parsley) or spices (like cumin) for better flavor.

3. Bulgur salad with vegetables

- Benefits: Bulgur has a moderate GI, but it remains relatively lower than other types of refined carbohydrates. It is rich in fiber and nutrients.
- Suggestions: Be sure to use a variety of fresh vegetables (like tomatoes, cucumbers, peppers and spinach) to maximize the vitamins and minerals in the salad. Avoid sweet sauces for seasoning.

4. Two little Swiss cheeses with arbutus compote

- Benefits: Petits suisses are an excellent source of protein and are relatively low in carbohydrates. Arbutus compote, if it is without added sugars, can provide a touch of sweetness while maintaining a low GI, because arbutus plants have a relatively low GI.
- Suggestions: If you are using a ready-made compote, check the label to make sure there are no added sugars. You can also make your own compote without sugar.

Conclusion

This meal seems well balanced with proteins, good fats and suitable carbohydrates, while being rich in vegetables. Just be sure to control portions and choose ingredients without added sugar to truly stay low GI. This should allow you to enjoy your meal in peace! Enjoy your food !

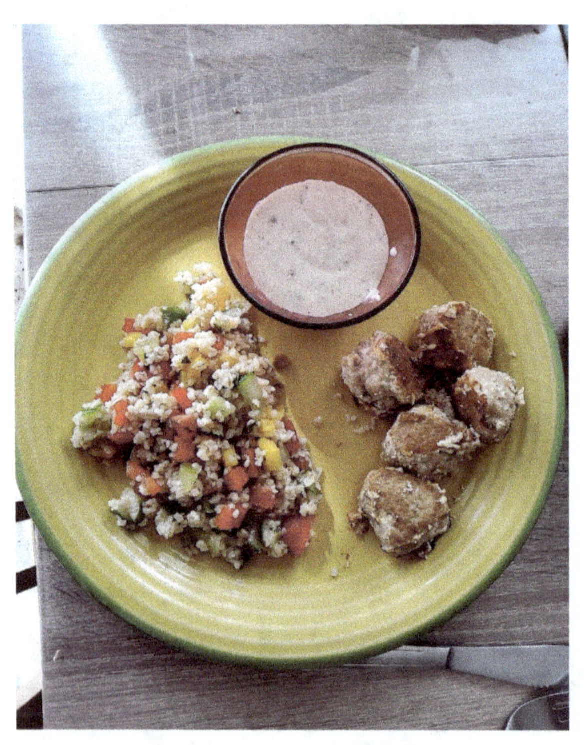